EMOTIONAL INTELLIGENCE

Cracking the Code for Men & Male Youth

CLARENCE J. GRANT, JR.

EMOTIONAL INTELLIGENCE

Cracking the Code for Men & Male Youth

CLARENCE J. GRANT, JR.

ISBN # 978-1-68593-234-3

Copyright © 2025

All rights reserved. No part of this book may be reproduced in any form or by any electronic or mechanical means including information storage and retrieval systems without permission in writing from the publisher, except by a reviewer, who may quote brief passages in a review.

Additional copies are available from the author, Clarence J. Grant, Jr.+

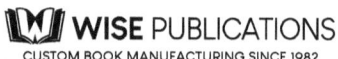

CUSTOM BOOK MANUFACTURING SINCE 1982

809 East Napoleon St., Sulphur, Louisiana 70663
337-527-8308 | wisepublications@yahoo.com
Visit our online Bookstore! www.wisepublications.biz

WAYS TO CONNECT

Email: info@theguytalkpod.com

Website: www.theguytalkpod.com

Instagram: @theguytalkpod

YouTube: The Guy Talk Pod

Facebook: The Guy Talk Pod

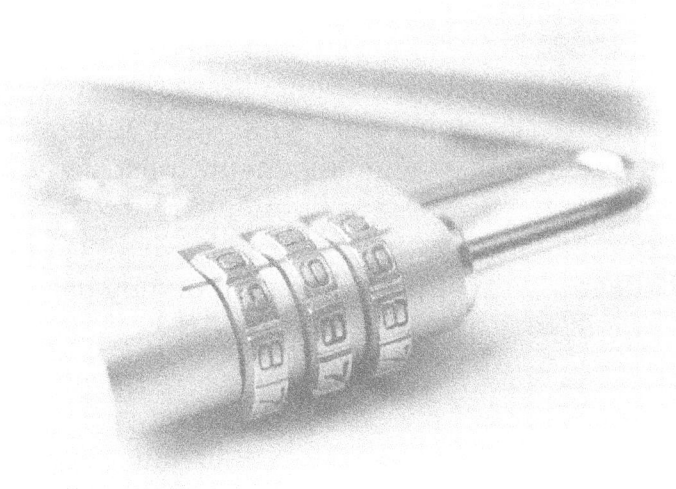

INTRODUCTION

Why Emotional Intelligence Is Your Superpower

Success is no longer determined by just how smart you are, the qualifications you hold, or the skills you've mastered. Beneath all of this, something even more vital shapes your path: your emotional intelligence (EI). Emotional Intelligence is the ability to recognize, understand, and handle your own emotions while connecting with those around you. Whether it's managing the pressure to succeed, staying calm in conflict, or building trust in relationships, EI often defines the strength, resilience, and authenticity that many men and young men never realize they possess. It's the hidden edge that can transform how you show up for yourself, your family, your team, and your community.

Emotional Intelligence isn't about suppressing or ignoring your emotions; it's about embracing them, understanding their purpose, and channeling them constructively. It's the difference between reacting impulsively to a situation and responding thoughtfully and calmly. It's the ability to connect deeply with others while maintaining balance and composure in your own life.

This book will serve as your guide and roadmap to mastering Emotional Intelligence, offering you the tools to navigate the depths of your emotions with clarity and purpose. It will challenge you to confront what you've suppressed, uncover the strength in vulnerability, and transform your emotions into powerful solutions for growth, connection, and fulfillment. Through this journey, you'll not only understand yourself more deeply but also discover how to live with intention, resilience, and impact.

Why Emotional Intelligence Matters

Emotional intelligence matters because it's the invisible thread weaving through every moment of our lives, shaping how we think, act, and connect with others. It's not just a skill; it's the foundation of how we navigate the world. For men and male youth, understanding and mastering emotional intelligence is about more than success or relationships; it's about survival, growth, and the legacy you leave behind.

> *In a world that often tells men and male youth to suppress what they feel, emotional intelligence offers freedom.*

Have you ever reacted in anger and regretted it later? Or felt misunderstood because you couldn't find the words to express what you were going through? These aren't random moments; they're signals. Signals that without emotional intelligence, we risk being prisoners of our own emotions. Emotions will always demand to be felt, but without awareness and control, they can drive us to make decisions that damage our relationships, derail our goals, and even hurt ourselves.

Emotional intelligence isn't about being soft or overly emotional. EI is about being strong enough to face what's inside you. It's about knowing that ignoring pain doesn't make it go away; it makes it fester. It's about understanding that avoiding a tough conversation doesn't solve the problem; it only prolongs the conflict. It's about realizing that success isn't just about what you achieve, but how you show up for the people who depend on you.

Think about the men you admire most. They aren't just strong, they're steady. They can stay calm when everything around them feels chaotic. They can lead with clarity because they understand themselves and the people they're guiding. They can take a hit—emotionally, physically, or mentally—and not let it define them. That's emotional intelligence. It's what separates those who crumble under pressure from those who rise above it.

For male youth, emotional intelligence is the key to breaking cycles. Cycles of anger, frustration, and regret. It gives you the tools to handle rejection without losing confidence, to face failure without feeling defeated, and to have meaningful conversations without fear of judgment. Emotional intelligence is what teaches you that strength isn't about never falling; it's about getting back up every single time.

In a world that often tells men and male youth to suppress what they feel, emotional intelligence offers freedom. Freedom to express yourself without shame, to build relationships that matter, and to face challenges without fear of breaking. It's not just important—it's urgent. Because without it, we risk losing not just who we are, but who we could become.

Emotional intelligence matters because it gives you the power to be in control; not of others, but of yourself. And when you master yourself, you can face anything. This isn't just about being better for others; it's about being the best version of you, for your family, your community, and most importantly, yourself. That's why emotional intelligence matters—because it's not just a skill to learn, but a way to live.

EMOTIONAL INTELLIGENCE

Cracking the Code for Men & Male Youth

WHO THIS BOOK IS FOR?

This book is for men who are ready to break free from the silent battles they fight within themselves, the struggles you may not even have words for. It's for the young men navigating the challenges of understanding who they are, their emotions, and relationships, in a world that often tells them to hide their feelings.

It's for the fathers striving to lead by example, showing their children that strength lies in vulnerability and growth. It's for the athletes who know that mastering their mental and emotional game is just as crucial as their physical training. For the men who carry the weight of expectations; whether at work, at home, or within themselves, and wonder, "How can I show up for the people and goals that I care about, when I don't know what to feel or how to express those feelings?"

> *This book is for men who are ready to break free from the silent battles they fight within themselves...*

This book will provide you more than just answers. It will offer solutions and a path to understanding your emotions—showing you that they aren't meant to be suppressed, but embraced as a source of strength, clarity, and wisdom. Through this journey, you'll uncover how to channel your emotions into building deeper relationships, finding peace within yourself, and creating a legacy of growth and impact for your family, children and all those that come in contact with you!

Now, let's dive into each chapter, and prepare you with the tools to transform your emotions into your greatest strength. As you read chapter to chapter, remember, Emotional Intelligence is YOUR SUPERPOWER! Now, let's Crack The Code!

EMOTIONAL INTELLIGENCE

Cracking the Code for Men & Male Youth

FOREWORD

There is a silent battle that many men and young men face every single day; the battle with their own emotions. Society has often conditioned men to be tough, to suppress their feelings, and to handle everything alone. But what if I told you that true strength isn't about hiding emotions, but mastering them?

That's exactly what *Emotional Intelligence: Cracking The Code for Men & Male Youth* is all about.

When Clarence Grant, Jr. first shared his vision for this book with me, I immediately understood why this message is needed now more than ever. As a pastor and youth leader, I've seen firsthand how the inability to process emotions can break relationships, limit opportunities, and keep men stuck in cycles of frustration and failure. Whether it's on the field, in the workplace, or at home, men who lack emotional intelligence struggle to communicate, struggle to lead, and struggle to thrive.

But God never designed us to be emotionally disconnected. Throughout Scripture, we see that wisdom, self-control, and understanding emotions are not just practical tools but spiritual principles. Proverbs 16:32 says, *"Better to be patient than powerful; better to have self-control than to conquer a city."* This reminds us that true strength is found not in force, but in the ability to manage our emotions with wisdom and patience.

What Clarence has done in this book is powerful. Instead of just talking about Emotional Intelligence as an abstract idea, he breaks it down in a real, relatable, and actionable way. He meets men and male youth where they are; whether they are athletes navigating pressure, young men building confidence, or fathers and leaders shaping the next generation.

This book isn't just about emotions. It's about understanding yourself, handling conflict, building stronger relationships, and developing the discipline needed to navigate life's highs and lows. It teaches that Emotional Intelligence is more than a skill, it's a blueprint for success in every area of life, including your spiritual walk.

One of the most valuable aspects of this book is its ability to tie Emotional Intelligence to faith. It reinforces the idea that God calls men to be wise, discerning, and emotionally grounded. Jesus Himself displayed the highest level of Emotional Intelligence, showing patience in conflict, empathy for others, and self-control in the face of betrayal and suffering. As men striving to become better, we are called to develop that same level of awareness and discipline.

What I love most about this book is that it doesn't just tell you *why* Emotional Intelligence is important; it shows you how to develop it. Through real-life examples, interactive reflections, and practical exercises, Clarence equips men with the tools they need to handle stress, lead with wisdom, and build a legacy that lasts.

If you've ever struggled to control your emotions, to communicate in difficult moments, or to become the best version of yourself in both life and faith, this book is for you.

It's time to crack the code.
— *Pastor Marcus Winfrey*

TABLE OF CONTENTS

Chapter 1: Emotional Intelligence 1

Chapter 2: Self Awareness 8

Chapter 3: Self Regulation 14

Chapter 4: Motivation 21

Chapter 5: Empathy 27

Chapter 6: Social Skills 32

Chapter 7: How Does EI Help with Conflict Resolution 37

Chapter 8: Current State of Emotional Intelligence 42

Chapter 9: Emotional Intelligence in Action 48

Chapter 10: The Emotional Game 52

Chapter 11: Leadership Beyond Authority 58

Chapter 12: Mastering the Moment 63

Chapter 13: What Does God Say About Emotional Intelligence .. 68

Chapter 14: EI Turns Mental Health Into Mental Wealth 73

Chapter 15: The Final Chapter, EI The First Choice 79

Final Message: The Legacy of Emotional Intelligence 85

From the Author 89

CHAPTER 1

"A rich man without control of his emotions is a prisoner of his own wealth, isolated by walls he cannot tear down. But a man who has mastered his emotions holds a treasure far greater; relationships, peace, and the ability to thrive in every area of his life."

- Clarence J. Grant, Jr.

Emotional Intelligence: The Foundation of Success

What is Emotional Intelligence? How can this ever make me successful? Why wasn't I ever taught this? Glad you asked!

Most of us grew up in environments where emotions weren't exactly a priority. Instead of being taught how to deal with what we feel, we were told to "man up" or "keep it moving." For many of us, vulnerability was seen as weakness, and showing emotion wasn't part of the playbook. This mindset has been passed down for generations, leaving us to figure it out on our own. But here's the thing; emotional intelligence is just as important as any skill you can learn in school or on the job. The fact that it wasn't taught to you isn't your fault, but it's on us now to change the narrative. This book is here to give you the tools to do just that and to show you that understanding your emotions IS NOT a weakness!

> *For generations, society has discouraged men and our male youth from openly expressing emotions...*

Emotional intelligence is the ability to recognize, understand, and manage your own emotions while effectively navigating and understanding the emotions of others. Simply put, emotional intelligence is about understanding your feelings, knowing how to manage them, and recognizing how they affect the way you interact with others. It's about staying in control when you're angry, expressing yourself without shutting down, and learning how to communicate in ways that strengthen your relationships.

For generations, society has discouraged men and our male youth from openly expressing emotions, equating being vulnerable, with weakness. This has led to emotional suppression, strained relationships, mental health challenges, and the inability to resolve conflicts. This can no longer be the norm to how men, fathers, sons, husbands, & male youth, view their emotions. And as of today, this changes for you!

How Does Emotional Intelligence Play a Role In My Success?

First, it's important to understand that Success isn't defined solely by talent, knowledge, or hard work— it's shaped by how you handle the challenges that life throws your way. When you ask yourself, "How does emotional intelligence play a role in my success?" Consider this: your ability to succeed starts with how well you understand and manage yourself and the relationships around you. Do you know a person who is highly talented, maybe even exceptionally knowledgeable in their field, but struggles to manage their emotions when faced with pressure or difficult conversations? Now, ask yourself, how likely are you to trust them with important decisions, follow their lead, or rely on them in critical moments? Emotional intelligence isn't just an advantage; it's what sets apart those who thrive under pressure from those who crumble.

For male youth, emotional intelligence is the skill that transforms potential into progress. It's what helps you calm your nerves before stepping onto the court or field during a big game. It allows you to focus and stay composed during a tough exam when your thoughts feel scattered. It gives you the confidence to stand up and speak in front of a group, even when your heart is racing. Emotional intelligence helps you find the words to express how you feel when you're frustrated with a friend

> *Emotional intelligence isn't just an advantage; it's what sets apart those who thrive under pressure from those who crumble.*

or upset at home, allowing you to resolve conflicts instead of letting them build.

> *Think about who you admire. Are they the ones who lose control when things go wrong?*

For men, emotional intelligence is the key to navigating the complexities of life and relationships. It's what helps you de-escalate an argument with your partner instead of letting tempers flare. It enables you to deliver constructive feedback to a team member at work without alienating them. It's the patience to guide your children through a difficult moment with understanding instead of frustration. Emotional intelligence is also what gives you the clarity to make tough decisions—whether in your career, your family, or your community—without letting fear or anger cloud your judgment.

Think about the men you admire. Are they the ones who lose control when things go wrong? Or are they the ones who stay composed, adapt, and find solutions? Emotional intelligence equips you to be the latter. It's the foundation of resilience, leadership, and respect, both from others and for yourself.

As we close this first chapter, remember that emotional intelligence is not just a skill, it's a transformative force that can redefine how you live, lead, and connect with others and yourself. The journey you've begun is about more than understanding your emotions; it's about unlocking the potential within you to shape your relationships, your decisions, and your future. This is just the beginning, and as we move forward, you'll discover that the power to reshape your life has always been within you. I hope you feel the chains breaking and now setting you free which will now allow for you to build a foundation for lasting success and fulfillment.

Tools for Men

1. **Daily Emotional Check-In**: Spend five minutes each morning reflecting on how you feel and what might be influencing your emotions. Awareness is the first step to mastery.

2. **Intentional Conversations**: Choose one conversation each day where you focus on actively listening and understanding the other person's emotions.

3. **Set a Personal Goal**: Identify one area in your life—relationships, career, or health—where you want to apply emotional intelligence. Track your progress weekly.

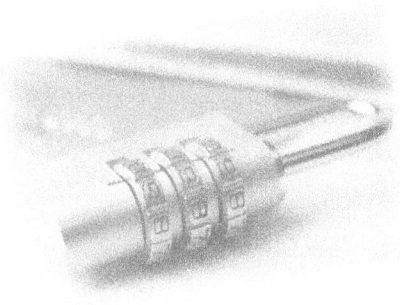

Tools for Male Youth

1. **Emotion Journal**: Write down three emotions you feel each day and what caused them. Over time, notice patterns and triggers.

2. **Find a Role Model**: Identify someone you admire who shows emotional intelligence and observe how they handle situations.

3. **Practice One New Habit**: Whether it's pausing before reacting or listening without interrupting, focus on practicing one EI habit for a week.

EMOTIONAL INTELLIGENCE

Cracking the Code for Men & Male Youth

Reflect & Journal

- *How do I currently handle my emotions?*
- *What role do I think emotional intelligence plays in my success?*
- *What actions can I take to better understand and manage my emotions?*

_____
_____
_____
_____
_____
_____
_____
_____
_____
_____
_____
_____
_____
_____
_____

Now, we will dive into the five essential components of emotional intelligence: self-awareness, self-regulation, motivation, empathy, and social skills. These are the building blocks that will guide you toward mastering your emotions and creating the life you've always envisioned. Let's keep going—your best self is waiting to emerge!

CHAPTER 2

"The first step toward change is awareness. The second step is acceptance."

— Nathaniel Branden

Self-Awareness: Knowing YourSelf

Self-awareness is understanding your emotions, strengths, weaknesses, values, and triggers. It's one of the foundational components of emotional intelligence allowing you to make informed decisions and respond thoughtfully.

Self-awareness is a major key to mastering your life. For men, it begins with asking the tough questions: *What drives me? What frustrates me? Why do I react the way I do in certain situations?* Too often, men are taught to power through their emotions, ignoring the signals their mind and body are sending. But self-awareness isn't about weakness—it's about strength. It's the ability to pause, reflect, and understand your own patterns, triggers, and values.

Imagine this: You're in a heated argument with your partner. The anger rises, and your instinct is to lash out or shut down. Self-awareness is what allows you to pause, recognize the anger for what it is, and ask yourself, *Why am I reacting this way? What's the real issue here?* That moment of reflection can transform a potential conflict into an opportunity for connection, understanding, and potentially save a friendship or marriage. For men, self-awareness isn't just about personal growth; it's about becoming the kind of man who leads with intention and earns respect, not because of dominance, but because of integrity and emotional clarity.

For male youth, self-awareness is like discovering a superpower you never knew you had. It's about recognizing what makes you unique—your strengths, your weaknesses, your emotions—and learning how to use that understanding to navigate life. Think about how often you feel frustrated at school, on the field, or even with friends. Have you ever stopped to ask yourself, *Why am I feeling this way? What's really going on inside me?*

Let's say you're struggling with a tough class. Instead of thinking, *I'm just not smart enough,* self-awareness helps you reframe it: *Maybe I'm overwhelmed, or maybe I need to approach this differently.* It's what gives you the ability to recognize when you need help and the courage to ask for it. Self-awareness is what keeps you grounded during the highs and steady during the lows, helping you avoid impulsive decisions that could hold you back. As a young man, learning to understand yourself now will prepare you

> *For male youth, self-awareness is like discovering a superpower you never knew you had.*

to face life's challenges with confidence, resilience, and a clear sense of who you are.

Let's look at another example. For many men, self-awareness around their health has not always been a priority. Too often, men avoid doctor visits, delay check-ups, or dismiss the warning signs their bodies are giving them. This lack of self-awareness has, in some cases, led to preventable illnesses or even untimely deaths. Ignoring your health doesn't make you stronger—it makes you vulnerable in ways you may not realize.

For both men and male youth, the path to true health starts with the ability to look inward, to listen to what your body and mind are telling you, and to act with intention. In a world that often teaches us to ignore pain, silence emotions, and push through without reflection, self-awareness should now become a necessary element of your life, for a better quality of life. It's the key to unlocking a healthier, stronger version of yourself, one that doesn't just survive but thrives.

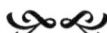

Recognizing your emotions, triggers, and patterns is only the first step.

The true power now lies in what you do with this understanding. Can you take what you've discovered about self-awareness, yourself and channel it into intentional, thoughtful action? Can you respond instead of react? This is where self-regulation comes in—the ability to take control of your emotions, rather than letting them control you.

As we move into the next chapter, we'll explore how self-regulation can help you turn reflection into resilience, impulsiveness into intention, and chaos into clarity. Together, these tools will prepare you to face life's challenges with confidence and composure. Let's continue building this foundation—your journey is only just beginning.

Tools for Men

1. **Mirror Exercise**: Stand in front of a mirror and describe what you feel in the moment. Name your emotions and reflect on why you feel them.

2. **Feedback Sessions**: Ask trusted friends or colleagues to share how they perceive your reactions in stressful situations. Use this to identify blind spots.

3. **Weekly Reflection**: At the end of each week, write down three situations where your emotions influenced your actions. Evaluate what you learned.

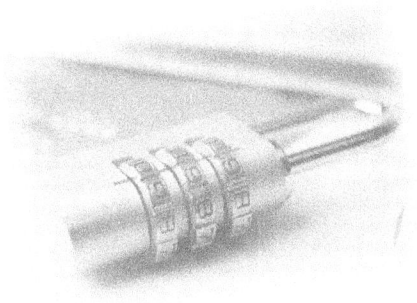

Tools for Male Youth

1. **Emotion Vocabulary**: Learn new words to describe how you feel (e.g., frustrated, disappointed, hopeful). Use them in your daily reflections.

2. **Self-Check Pause**: Throughout the day, pause and ask yourself, "What am I feeling right now, and why?"

3. **Strengths and Challenges List**: Write down three strengths you have and three areas where you struggle emotionally. Reflect on how to improve.

EMOTIONAL INTELLIGENCE
Cracking the Code for Men & Male Youth

Reflect & Journal

- *What emotions or triggers am I most aware of in my daily life?*
- *How can self-awareness help me navigate difficult situations?*
- *What steps can I take to build my self-awareness?*

_____
_____
_____
_____
_____
_____
_____
_____
_____
_____
_____
_____
_____
_____
_____
_____
_____
_____
_____

CHAPTER 3

But the Holy Spirit produces this kind of fruit in our lives: love, joy, peace, patience, kindness, goodness, faithfulness, gentleness, and **Self-Control.** *There is no law against these things!"*

— *Galatians 5:22-23 (NLT)*

Self-Regulation: Mastering Emotional Control

Self-regulation involves managing your emotions, especially in stressful or triggering situations, and behaving in ways that align with your values.

Self-regulation is the bridge between self-awareness and intentional action. As men, we are often taught that strength is about control; control over situations, people, or outcomes. But true strength lies in the ability to control yourself: your emotions, your impulses, and your reactions. Think about the last time you faced frustration at work or an argument at home. Did you react immediately, fueled by anger or pride? Or did you take a moment to pause, reflect, and respond with intention?

Self-regulation isn't about suppressing how you feel; it's about channeling those emotions constructively. For example, when a deadline is missed or a deal falls apart, the impulse might be to lash out or assign blame. But self-regulation allows you to step back, evaluate the situation objectively, and choose a response that fosters solutions instead of conflict. It's what helps you remain steady when the people around you are losing control, and it's what earns respect as someone who can lead under pressure. Mastering self-regulation doesn't just make you a better man—it makes you the kind of man others trust to guide them through chaos.

For male youth, self-regulation is the difference between acting on impulse and taking control of your choices. In the heat of the moment;whether it's during a game, an argument with a friend, a conflict at home, or conflict in our communities, it's easy to let emotions take over. Maybe you've said something out of anger that you wish you could take back, or you've made a choice in frustration that led to regret. Self-regulation is about learning to pause, breathe, and think before you act.

> *Self-regulation isn't about suppressing how you feel; it's about channeling those emotions constructively.*

Imagine you're on the basketball court, and the referee makes a bad call. The impulse is to argue or lose focus, but self-regulation helps you stay composed, channeling that energy into your performance instead of letting frustration derail or distract you. It's about understanding that while you can't always control what happens around you, you can always control how you respond. When you master this skill, you don't just gain control over your emotions; you gain control over your life. Self-regulation gives you the tools to handle challenges with maturity and confidence, preparing you for the responsibilities ahead.

Self Regulation Example: David, a young father, finds himself snapping at his kids after long workdays. Recognizing the pattern, he implements a "ten-minute rule," taking ten minutes to decompress before engaging with his family. Over time, this small change significantly improves their relationship.

Self-regulation may very well be the most important component of emotional intelligence. It's here where the true weight of our choices is revealed—where the inability to manage emotions can lead to broken relationships, conflicts that escalate into violence, health issues fueled by unchecked stress, and decisions driven by greed or impulse. Without self-regulation, emotions like anger, jealousy, and fear can take over, turning momentary reactions into lasting consequences.

> *Self-regulation may very well be the most important component of emotional intelligence.*

Think about how many families have been torn apart by unresolved arguments, how many communities have been scarred by crime born out of conflict, and how many lives have been lost because someone couldn't pause long enough to think before acting. The absence of self-regulation doesn't just impact you—it ripples outward, affecting your family, your relationships, and the people who look up to you.

For men, self-regulation is the difference between leading with wisdom and reacting with recklessness. It's the discipline to walk away from a heated exchange, the courage to admit when you're wrong, and the strength to respond thoughtfully even when emotions run high. For male youth, self-regulation is a skill that will shape the course of your future—teaching you how to handle setbacks, resolve conflicts, and make decisions that build a life of integrity and purpose.

> *The lack of self-regulation can lead to destruction, but mastering it can lead to transformation.*

The lack of self-regulation can lead to destruction, but mastering it can lead to transformation. It's not just about keeping your emotions in check—it's about choosing a life of peace, stability, and strength for yourself, your family, and your community. This is why self-regulation is not just a skill—it's a responsibility.

Self-regulation is the key to navigating life with clarity and purpose. It gives you the ability to take control of your emotions, guiding them instead of being controlled by them. It's what allows you to remain calm in the face of chaos, to turn anger into understanding, and to transform frustration into action. But self-regulation isn't just about restraint—it's about living in alignment with the Spirit. As Galatians 5:22-23 reminds us, self-control is a fruit of the Spirit, a sign of God working within us to bring peace, patience, and gentleness into every area of our lives.

When we invite God into our process of self-regulation, we find strength that goes beyond our own understanding. Through prayer and reflection, we gain the ability to pause, reflect, and choose a response that honors both our values and God's purpose for us.

As we move into the next chapter, we'll explore the driving force that keeps you moving forward: motivation. If self-regulation helps you stay grounded, motivation is what helps you rise. It's the fuel that turns obstacles into opportunities and setbacks into stepping stones. Together, these tools will not only shape how you respond to the world but also how you achieve the life God has called you to live. Let's keep building—your journey is far from over.

Tools for Men

1. **The Pause Method**: When faced with a triggering situation, take a deep breath and count to ten before responding. This creates space for thoughtful action.

2. **Personal Cool-Down Routine**: Develop a routine (e.g., listening to calming music, going for a walk) that helps you regain composure in stressful moments.

3. **Mindful Reframing**: When faced with a setback, reframe it by asking, "What can I learn from this?" instead of focusing on the loss.

Tools for Male Youth

1. **Deep Breathing Exercise**: Practice a simple technique: Inhale for four seconds, hold for four seconds, and exhale for six seconds. Use this whenever you feel overwhelmed.

2. **"I" Statements**: When upset, practice expressing yourself by starting sentences with "I feel..." instead of blaming others. For example, "I feel upset because I wasn't included."

3. **Impulse Tracker**: Write down situations where you acted impulsively. Reflect on what triggered the reaction and what you could do differently next time.

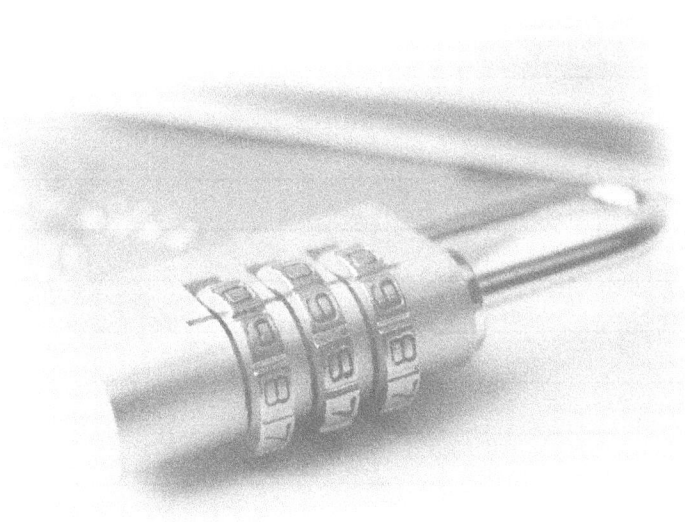

Reflect & Journal

- *How do I currently manage my emotions under stress?*
- *What specific strategies could I use to improve my self-regulation?*
- *Reflect on a time you successfully controlled an emotional response—what worked?*

_____
_____
_____
_____
_____
_____
_____
_____
_____
_____
_____
_____
_____
_____
_____
_____
_____

CHAPTER 4

"Motivation isn't found in the absence of challenges; it's born in the way you rise to meet them. Every step within that challenge, strengthens the foundation of who you are becoming."

Motivation: Fueling Your Inner Drive

Motivation is the driving force behind every achievement, but for many men, it's easy to lose sight of what truly fuels you. Society often teaches men that motivation should come from external rewards—success, status, or financial gain. But true motivation runs deeper. It comes from knowing your purpose, aligning your actions with your values, and pushing forward even when the road is difficult.

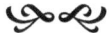

Think about the times you've faced setbacks. Maybe it was a failed business, a tough season in your marriage, or a personal goal that seemed impossible to reach. What kept you going? Motivation isn't just about ambition—it's about resilience. It's what helps you wake up each day and give your best, even when no one is watching. For men, motivation is the ability to look beyond the obstacles and keep your eyes fixed on the bigger picture. It's what helps you lead your family, serve your community, and strive for greatness not because others demand it, but because you demand it of yourself.

> *Motivation isn't a constant; it's a practice.*

Motivation isn't a constant; it's a practice. It requires discipline, self-reflection, and faith in what's possible. When you're connected to your purpose, you'll find that motivation isn't something you need to search for—it becomes part of who you are.

EMOTIONAL INTELLIGENCE
Cracking the Code for Men & Male Youth

Tools for Motivation:

1. **Write Down Your Why**: Take 5 minutes to write down why your goals matter. Keep this list visible as a daily reminder.

2. **Set Small, Achievable Goals**: Break large goals into smaller steps. Celebrate each accomplishment to build momentum.

3. **Surround Yourself with Accountability**: Share your goals with someone you trust and ask them to check in with you regularly.

4. **Visualize Success**: Spend a few minutes each day imagining how achieving your goal will feel and look.

5. **Practice Gratitude**: Reflect daily on three things you're grateful for. Gratitude fuels positive energy and keeps you focused on growth.

For male youth, motivation is what turns dreams into action. It's what gives you the drive to push through challenges at school, on the field, or in your personal life. At this stage, it's easy to feel overwhelmed by obstacles or to give up when something feels too hard. But motivation is about more than just finishing the race—it's about finding the reason why you started in the first place.

Imagine you're struggling with a class you don't understand, a sport where you feel you're falling behind, or a goal that feels out of reach. Motivation is the voice inside you that says, *Keep going.* It's not about being the best; it's about becoming better than you were yesterday. Maybe you're driven by the dream of creating a better life for your family, proving to yourself that you can succeed, or inspiring others around you. Whatever it is, motivation is what helps you push through discomfort, stay focused, and take one step closer to the person you want to be.

Let me be very clear and honest with you, motivation isn't always easy. This journey will require effort, determination, and a belief that your hard work will pay off. But when you embrace it, you'll find that the challenges in front of you are no match for the strength within you. This will be the spark that ignites action, but it will be the consistency of that action that creates lasting change.

As you move forward, remember that motivation isn't always loud or obvious; it's often the quiet resolve to keep going when the road gets tough. It's rooted in your purpose, your values, and the vision you hold for your life. When challenges arise, let your motivation remind you why you started and who you're becoming.

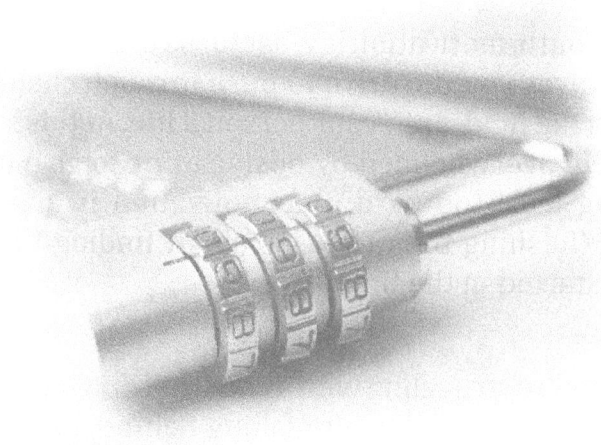

Tools for Motivation:

1. **Set a Daily Goal**: Choose one thing to accomplish each day. Completing small goals builds confidence for larger challenges.

2. **Track Your Progress**: Keep a journal or checklist of your progress to see how far you've come.

3. **Find Role Models**: Identify someone you admire and study how they overcame challenges. Use their story as inspiration.

4. **Reward Yourself**: Celebrate small wins by treating yourself to something you enjoy, like a favorite meal or activity.

5. **Focus on Effort, Not Perfection**: Remind yourself that trying and improving is more important than being perfect.

Reflect & Journal

- *What is my "why"? What motivates me to keep going when things get tough, and how do I stay connected to it?*

- *How do I handle setbacks or failures? Do I allow them to stop me, or do I find ways to learn and move forward?*

- *What habits or daily practices can I implement to keep my motivation strong and consistent?*

_____
_____
_____
_____
_____
_____
_____
_____
_____
_____

Now, as we move into the next chapter on empathy, we'll explore the power of understanding and connection—a critical component in building meaningful relationships and thriving in every area of life. Let's continue shaping the person you're meant to be. You've come too far to turn around!!

CHAPTER 5

"Empathy is not about fixing others' pain; it's about sharing in it, so no one has to face it alone. Its the ability to understand and share the feelings of others and recognizing that it's not always a voice someone needs, sometimes, it's just an ear they need"

Empathy: Connecting Through Understanding

Empathy is the ability to step outside your own perspective and truly understand the emotions and experiences of others. For many men, empathy may feel like a vulnerability, something that society has discouraged in the name of toughness. But in reality, empathy is one of the most powerful tools a man can possess. It allows you to connect deeply with your partner, your children, your coworkers, and your community.

Think about the last time someone confided in you. Were you fully present, or were you thinking of how to solve the problem or respond? Empathy is about listening—not to reply, but to understand. It's the strength to see someone's pain without judgment and to offer support without needing to fix everything. For men, empathy is what transforms relationships from surface-level interactions to bonds built on trust and respect. It's what allows you to lead with compassion, parent with patience, and love with intention.

> ## Tools for Men:
>
> 1. **Practice Active Listening**: Put away distractions, make eye contact, and focus entirely on what the other person is saying. Repeat back what you've heard to confirm understanding.
>
> 2. **Ask Open-Ended Questions**: Encourage deeper conversations by asking questions like, "How are you feeling about that?" or "What can I do to support you?"
>
> 3. **Reflect on Your Own Experiences**: Think about a time when you needed understanding. Use that memory to relate to others.

For male youth, empathy is a skill that helps you navigate friendships, family relationships, and even conflicts. It's what allows you to understand what others are going through, even when their experiences are different from your own. Empathy helps you be the kind of friend who others can trust and the kind of person who can build connections that last.

Imagine a friend at school who seems distant or upset. Instead of ignoring it or assuming it's not your business, empathy encourages you to reach out and ask, "Are you okay?" It's not about having all the answers; it's about showing you care. Empathy also helps you handle conflict by seeing the situation from the other person's perspective, which can turn arguments into opportunities for understanding. As a young man, learning empathy now will set you apart, helping you form stronger friendships and relationships as you grow.

> ## Tools for Male Youth:
>
> 1. **Put Yourself in Someone Else's Shoes**: When a friend or family member is upset, imagine how you'd feel in their situation.
>
> 2. **Check In with Others**: If you notice someone struggling, ask them how they're doing or offer to help.
>
> 3. **Practice Small Acts of Kindness**: Show empathy through actions like holding the door, offering a kind word, or simply being present for someone in need.

I hope that you have learned and understood that Empathy is the foundation of connection. This is what allows you to truly see, hear, and understand the people around you. It's a skill that strengthens relationships, resolves conflicts, and builds bridges where walls once stood. As you reflect on this chapter, remember that empathy is not just about feeling for others, it's about standing with them, offering compassion, and choosing understanding over judgment.

In the next chapter, we'll explore social skills; the tools that turn empathy into action and help you navigate relationships with confidence and intention. Let's keep building the skills that will transform your life and the lives of those around you. You're almost there!

EMOTIONAL INTELLIGENCE

Cracking the Code for Men & Male Youth

Reflect & Journal

- *How often do I listen to others without thinking about how I'll respond? What changes can I make to become a better listener?*

- *When was the last time I truly empathize with someone's situation, and how did it impact our relationship?*

- *How can developing empathy help me strengthen my relationships at home, work, or in my community?*

_____
_____
_____
_____
_____
_____
_____
_____
_____
_____
_____
_____
_____
_____
_____
_____

CHAPTER 6

"The most underrated social skill isn't talking to be heard, but listening to understand. True connection begins when we seek to understand, not just to reply."

— *Clarence J. Grant, Jr.*

Social Skills: Building Meaningful Connections

Social skills are the glue that holds relationships together, both personally and professionally. For men, mastering social skills means more than just being able to hold a conversation; it's about fostering trust, building rapport, and navigating conflict with grace. Strong social skills allow you to create deeper connections, lead with confidence, and influence those around you in meaningful ways.

Think about a time when a misunderstanding caused tension at work or at home. Did you address it directly, or let it fester? Social skills, like clear communication and active listening, are the tools that allow you to resolve conflicts before they escalate. They also help you build respect and camaraderie in your relationships. Whether you're leading a team, raising a family, or simply strengthening friendships, social skills are what set great leaders apart—they're the bridge between intention and impact.

> ## Tools for Men:
>
> 1. **Practice Nonverbal Communication**: Be aware of your body language, eye contact, and tone of voice—they often speak louder than words.
>
> 2. **Use "I" Statements**: In conflict, express your feelings without placing blame. For example, say, "I felt hurt when..." instead of "You always..."
>
> 3. **Focus on Solutions**: In tough conversations, steer the focus toward resolving the issue rather than dwelling on the problem.

For male youth, social skills are the tools that help you navigate school, friendships, and family dynamics. At this stage in life, learning how to communicate effectively can set you apart and give you the confidence to handle any situation. Social skills aren't just about being outgoing—they're about knowing when to speak, when to listen, and how to connect with others in a way that builds trust and respect.

Imagine you're working on a group project at school, and not everyone is contributing equally. Do you stay silent and let frustration build, or do you address the issue respectfully? Social skills give you the confidence to speak up, the tact to express yourself without creating conflict, and the leadership to guide others toward a solution. Whether you're making new friends, standing up for yourself, or resolving a disagreement, social skills are your key to success.

Tools for Male Youth:

1. **Ask Open-Ended Questions**: Show interest in others by asking questions like, "What do you think about this?" or "How did that make you feel?"

2. **Practice Small Talk**: Build confidence in casual conversations by starting with simple topics like hobbies or shared experiences.

3. **Learn to Apologize**: If you make a mistake, own it and say, "I'm sorry." It shows maturity and builds respect.

Social skills are more than just tools for communication—they're the foundation for building trust, resolving conflicts, and creating meaningful connections. They are what allow you to navigate relationships with confidence, inspire those around you, and leave a lasting positive impact wherever you go. As you reflect on this chapter, remember that social skills aren't just about what you say, but how you make others feel.

Now, as we move into the next chapter, we'll explore how emotional intelligence helps with one of life's most challenging aspects: conflict resolution. This is where your ability to understand and connect with others will truly be put to the test.

EMOTIONAL INTELLIGENCE

Cracking the Code for Men & Male Youth

Reflect & Journal

- *How do you handle social interactions when you feel uncomfortable? What can you improve?*

- *Think of a recent disagreement. How could better listening or patience have changed the outcome?*

- *What is one social skill you want to strengthen? What's a small step you can take today?*

CHAPTER 7

"Peace is not the absence of conflict, but the ability to handle conflict by peaceful means."

— Ronald Reagan

How Does EI Help with Conflict Resolution?

Conflict is a part of life; it arises in the workplace, at home, and even within yourself. For men, handling conflict effectively requires more than strength or dominance; it requires emotional intelligence. EI helps you approach disagreements not as battles to be won but as opportunities for growth and understanding.

Imagine a heated argument with a coworker or a partner. The instinct might be to defend yourself or to prove your point. But emotional intelligence teaches you to pause, assess the situation, and respond instead of reacting. By staying calm and seeking to understand the other person's perspective, you can de-escalate tension and find a resolution that benefits everyone involved. Mastering conflict resolution isn't about avoiding tough conversations, it's about approaching them with empathy, clarity, and respect.

> ## Tools for Men:
>
> 1. **Pause and Breathe**: Before responding, take a deep breath to calm your emotions and gather your thoughts.
>
> 2. **Seek to Understand**: Ask questions to clarify the other person's perspective, such as, "Can you help me understand what's bothering you?"
>
> 3. **Focus on the Solution**: Shift the conversation from assigning blame to finding common ground.

For male youth, conflict often feels overwhelming. Whether it's a disagreement with a friend, tension at home, or challenges at school, it's easy to let emotions take over. But emotional intelligence gives you the tools to navigate conflict with maturity and understanding.

Imagine you've had a falling-out with a teammate. Instead of arguing or holding a grudge, emotional intelligence helps you approach the situation calmly. You might say, "I felt upset when this happened, but I want us to work through it." Conflict resolution is not about proving who's right—it's about maintaining respect and strengthening relationships. Learning to handle conflict now will set you apart as a leader among your peers and prepare you for the challenges of adulthood.

> ## Tools for Male Youth:
>
> 1. **Use "I" Statements**: Express how you feel without blaming others. For example, "I felt hurt when you said that" instead of "You always insult me."
>
> 2. **Take a Break if Needed**: If emotions are running high, step away from the situation to cool down before addressing it.
>
> 3. **Look for Compromise**: Focus on what you can both agree on instead of dwelling on your differences.

When emotional intelligence is absent during conflict, the consequences can impact every area of your life; i.e. relationships, careers, health, and communities. Without the ability to regulate emotions, conflicts escalate quickly, turning minor disagreements into major divisions. In personal relationships, unresolved conflicts often lead to broken trust, resentment, and even the end of partnerships that once held great potential. A single argument left unaddressed can fester, creating emotional distance that's difficult to repair.

In the workplace, the inability to manage conflict constructively can derail teamwork, reduce productivity, and tarnish reputations. Leaders who react with anger or defensiveness instead of empathy and clarity lose the respect of their teams, while employees who avoid conflict altogether miss opportunities to resolve issues and build collaboration. The cost of unaddressed or poorly handled conflict can be felt in every missed promotion, strained working relationship, or toxic work environment.

For male youth, the stakes are equally high. Without emotional intelligence, conflicts in school or with peers can lead to damaged friendships, bullying, or isolation. Anger or frustration left unchecked can result in impulsive decisions—ones that could carry lifelong consequences, like strained relationships with parents or even encounters with legal trouble.

> *The cost of ignoring emotional intelligence is far greater than the effort it takes to develop and apply it.*

At a broader level, the lack of conflict resolution skills has a devastating impact on communities. Unresolved disputes can fuel cycles of violence, perpetuate misunderstandings, and erode the sense of unity and trust that hold societies together. Conflict is inevitable, but when emotional intelligence isn't present, its outcomes often leave wounds that linger far beyond the moment.

Failing to use emotional intelligence in conflict resolution isn't just about losing an argument or having a bad day—it's about the long-term damage that occurs when we let emotions dictate our actions instead of guiding them with clarity and purpose. The cost of ignoring emotional intelligence is far greater than the effort it takes to develop and apply it.

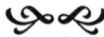

Reflect & Journal

- *How do I typically respond to conflict? Do I react impulsively, avoid it altogether, or approach it with a mindset of understanding and resolution?*

- *Think about a recent conflict in your life—what was the outcome, and how might using emotional intelligence have changed it?*

- *What steps can I take to better manage my emotions and improve my ability to resolve conflicts in my personal relationships, workplace, or community?*

_____
_____
_____
_____
_____
_____
_____
_____
_____
_____
_____
_____
_____
_____
_____
_____
_____

CHAPTER 8

Current State of Emotional Intelligence in Men & Male Youth

The current state of emotional intelligence in men and male youth is a reflection of the narratives society has reinforced for generations. Many men have grown up believing that emotional expression is a weakness, equating vulnerability with failure and silence with strength. This mindset has left countless men emotionally disconnected—not just from others, but from themselves. For male youth, these lessons are often absorbed early, shaping their understanding of masculinity in ways that limit their ability to process emotions, form healthy relationships, and face life's challenges with resilience.

> *Men who suppress their emotions are more likely to experience mental health struggles such as depression and anxiety.*

This emotional disconnect has consequences that ripple through every facet of life. Men who suppress their emotions are more likely to experience mental health struggles such as depression and anxiety. Relationships suffer when emotions are bottled up and communication breaks down. Male youth often act out their frustrations through aggression or withdrawal because they lack the tools to articulate what they're feeling. Without emotional intelligence, men and boys are left navigating a world that demands strength without equipping them to understand what true strength looks like.

Yet, despite these challenges, there is hope. Emotional intelligence is not innate—it is learned and developed. Men and male youth who take the time to cultivate self-awareness, empathy, and emotional control can break the cycle of emotional suppression. They can become better fathers, leaders, and friends. They can show the world that strength is not the absence of emotion, but the ability to face it with courage and clarity.

The current state of emotional intelligence in men and boys is a call to action. It's a challenge to unlearn what no longer serves us and to embrace the tools that lead to healthier, more fulfilling lives. The journey may not be easy, but the rewards are undeniable. By prioritizing emotional growth, men and male youth can redefine masculinity for themselves and future generations—creating a legacy of strength built on understanding, connection, and purpose.

Emotional intelligence is more than a concept—it's a measurable factor that impacts every aspect of life, from mental health to professional success. The numbers don't lie: the lack of emotional awareness and expression among men and male youth has real and far-reaching consequences. Consider these eye-opening statistics as a reminder of why prioritizing emotional intelligence is not just important—it's essential.

- **Self-Awareness Gap**: While 95% of people believe they are self-aware, only 10–15% actually are.
  Soocial

- **Mental Health Impact**: Men are less likely to seek help for mental health issues, often due to societal norms discouraging emotional expression. This reluctance contributes to higher rates of untreated mental health disorders among men.
  ADAA

- **Suicide Rates**: Globally, men have higher suicide rates compared to women, underscoring the severe consequences of emotional suppression.
  Boys Mentoring Advocacy Network

- **Workplace Performance**: Emotional intelligence accounts for 58% of job performance, and 90% of top performers have high EI. Despite this, many men may not fully develop EI skills due to traditional gender norms.
  Soocial

These statistics highlight the pressing need for men and male youth to cultivate emotional intelligence, not only for personal well-being but also for professional success and overall mental health.

Tools for Men

1. **Challenge the Narrative**: Reflect on the beliefs you've been taught about emotions and masculinity. Ask yourself if they serve you or hold you back.

2. **Practice Emotional Labeling**: Start identifying and naming your emotions to build self-awareness. For example, instead of saying, "I'm angry," explore whether it's frustration, disappointment, or hurt.

3. **Seek Mentorship or Counseling**: Connect with someone who can guide you through emotional challenges, whether it's a mentor, coach, or therapist.

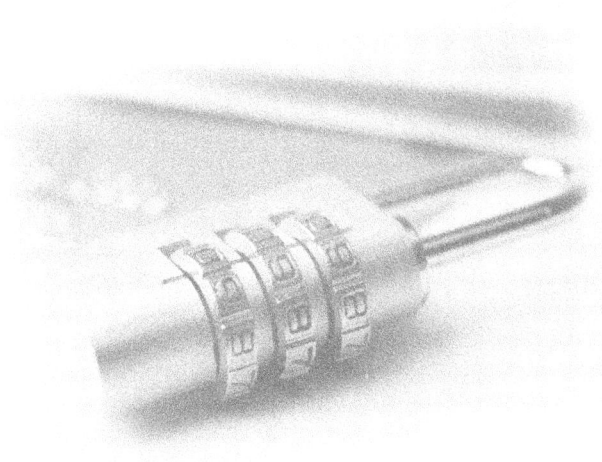

Tools for Male Youth

1. **Journaling Emotions**: Spend a few minutes each day writing about how you feel and what might have caused those emotions. This helps develop emotional awareness.

2. **Learn to Pause**: Practice pausing before reacting in heated situations. Count to ten or take a deep breath to process emotions.

3. **Role Models of Emotional Strength**: Identify and study men who exemplify emotional intelligence, whether they're family members, teachers, or public figures.

EMOTIONAL INTELLIGENCE

Cracking the Code for Men & Male Youth

Reflect & Journal

- *How have societal messages about masculinity shaped the way I express or suppress my emotions?*

- *What are some specific ways emotional suppression has impacted my relationships, health, or goals?*

- *What steps can I take today to begin building my emotional intelligence and redefine my understanding of strength?*

_____
_____
_____
_____
_____
_____
_____
_____
_____
_____
_____
_____
_____
_____
_____
_____
_____
_____
_____

CHAPTER 9

"The true measure of growth isn't what you know, but how you apply it. Emotional intelligence is your superpower; the bridge between who you are and who you're becoming."

- Clarence J. Grant, Jr.

Emotional Intelligence in Action: Your Next Steps

Emotional intelligence is not just a concept to understand—it's a way of living that transforms how you approach every area of your life. The knowledge you've gained throughout this book is only the beginning. What matters now is how you apply it. Emotional intelligence is a practice, and it's in the consistent action of using these principles that you unlock their true power. This chapter isn't about perfection; it's about progress. Your next steps are about taking what you've learned and making it a part of who you are.

For men, emotional intelligence in action means stepping into your relationships with intentionality. It's about being present for your partner, showing up for your children, and engaging with your friends in meaningful ways. It means leading at work with empathy, resolving conflicts with integrity, and having the courage to admit when you're wrong. It's about recognizing that strength is not measured by how much you can suppress, but by how willing you are to grow and connect. These steps won't just change how others see you—they'll change how you see yourself.

> *For men, emotional intelligence in action means stepping into your relationships with intentionality.*

For male youth, your next steps are about building a foundation for the man you want to become. Emotional intelligence will guide you as you navigate school, friendships, and family dynamics. It will give you the tools to face rejection with resilience, handle conflict with maturity, and build confidence in your ability to overcome challenges. Each step forward brings you closer to understanding your emotions, your values, and your potential. What you practice now will shape the man you'll become tomorrow.

Emotional intelligence in action also means making a commitment to consistency. There will be moments when it feels easier to revert to old habits—to lash out in anger, to avoid a hard conversation, or to ignore how you're feeling. But each time you choose to pause, reflect, and respond intentionally, you're building a stronger foundation. These small, intentional acts are what lead to long-term transformation.

The ripple effect of your actions extends beyond yourself. By living with emotional intelligence, you create environments where others feel safe, respected, and valued. You set an example for those around you, whether it's your family, your coworkers, or your peers. Emotional intelligence isn't just a personal journey—it's a legacy you leave in the lives you touch.

Your next steps are about living what you've learned. It's about showing up every day as the best version of yourself, knowing that the effort you put in today will shape your tomorrow. Emotional intelligence isn't just something you practice—it's something you become. Let this journey be a starting point, not an end. The next chapter of your life is waiting for you to write it with intention, courage, and purpose.

EMOTIONAL INTELLIGENCE

Cracking the Code for Men & Male Youth

Reflect & Journal

As you prepare to put emotional intelligence into action, take a moment to reflect on the journey you've undertaken. Your growth begins with self-awareness but extends into every decision, relationship, and opportunity you encounter. Use these questions to evaluate where you are and define how you will carry these lessons forward.

- *What are the specific areas of my life where I can start applying emotional intelligence immediately, and what steps will I take to do so?*

- *When faced with challenges or setbacks, how can I remind myself to pause, reflect, and respond with intention rather than reacting impulsively?*

- *What legacy do I want to leave for my family, friends, and community through the way I practice emotional intelligence in my daily life?*

_____
_____
_____
_____
_____
_____
_____
_____
_____
_____
_____

CHAPTER 10

"You can't always control circumstances. However, you can always control your attitude, approach, and response."

— Tony Dungy

> **The Emotional Game:**
> **How Emotional Intelligence**
> **Drives Athletic Excellence**

For men, sports can be more than a game—it's often a proving ground for discipline, teamwork, and leadership. But the unseen battles aren't fought on the field; they're fought within. Emotional intelligence (EI) is what allows you to master those battles. It's the ability to channel frustration into focus, to lead with clarity under pressure, and to remain composed in the face of setbacks. Without it, the weight of competition can lead to rash decisions, strained relationships, and self-doubt that impacts far beyond the game.

Imagine being the captain of a team during a championship game. The score is tight, and tensions are high. A teammate makes a critical error, and the natural impulse might be to lash out or express frustration. But emotional intelligence teaches you to pause, understand the moment, and respond constructively. Instead of blaming your teammate, you use words that build their confidence and rally the team. That's the power of emotional intelligence—it transforms moments of conflict into opportunities for growth and connection.

In the heat of competition, EI allows you to separate your emotions from your actions. It gives you the strength to focus on the solution instead of the problem. And it's not just about what happens during the game—it's about how you process the outcome afterward. Whether you win or lose, emotional intelligence equips you to reflect on your performance with honesty and use it as fuel for

For male youth, sports are often where you first encounter the lessons of resilience, teamwork, and discipline. But beyond the physical challenges, emotional intelligence is the skill that will set you apart. It's what helps you recover from a missed shot, stay focused when the game doesn't go your way, and be the kind of teammate others respect and rely on. Emotional intelligence isn't about ignoring your emotions—it's about understanding them and using them to your advantage.

> *Emotional intelligence teaches you to pause, understand the moment, and respond constructively.*

Imagine being benched during an important game. The initial reaction might be anger, frustration, or even embarrassment. Without emotional intelligence, those emotions can take over, causing you to disengage or lash out. But EI helps you step back and see the bigger picture. You realize that instead of reacting, you can use the time to observe, reflect, and prepare to contribute when your opportunity comes. This shift in mindset not only helps you grow as a player but also earns the respect of your coach and teammates.

> *Emotional intelligence also plays a role in how you handle your relationships on and off the field.*

Emotional intelligence also plays a role in how you handle your relationships on and off the field. When you understand how your words and actions affect others, you can become a leader who inspires and uplifts. Whether it's comforting a teammate after a tough loss or resolving a disagreement during practice, EI helps you navigate the emotional dynamics of sports with maturity and grace. Developing this skill now will prepare you not just for athletic success, but for life's challenges beyond the game.

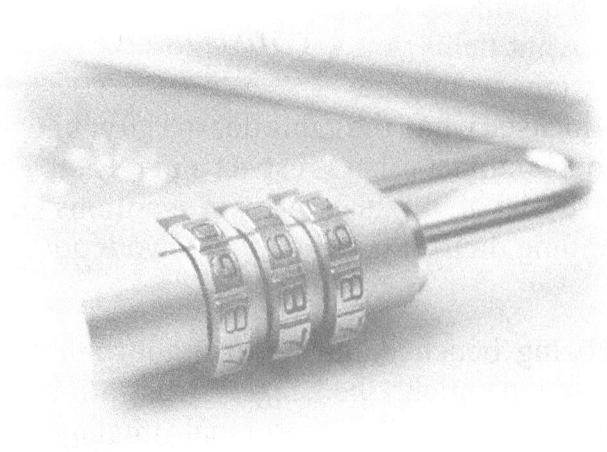

Tools for Men

1. **Emotion Check-Ins**: Before and after a game, take a moment to identify what you're feeling. Labeling emotions like frustration or excitement can help you manage them effectively.

2. **Visualization**: Spend time visualizing yourself handling high-pressure situations with calm and focus. This mental practice builds emotional resilience.

3. **Supportive Leadership**: Practice responding to mistakes—yours or others'—with encouragement instead of criticism. This builds trust and morale among teammates.

EMOTIONAL INTELLIGENCE

Cracking the Code for Men & Male Youth

Tools for Male Youth

1. **Game Reflection Journal**: After each practice or game, write about one thing you did well and one thing you can improve. Reflecting on your emotions helps you grow.

2. **Breathing Exercises**: Use deep breathing techniques to calm nerves before big moments, like free throws or penalty kicks. This keeps you focused under pressure.

3. **Empathy in Action**: Practice being aware of how your teammates might feel during stressful situations. Ask yourself, "How can I support them right now?"

EMOTIONAL INTELLIGENCE
Cracking the Code for Men & Male Youth

Reflect & Journal

- *Think of a time when emotions impacted your performance in sports. How did you handle it, and what could you do differently next time?*

- *How do you currently communicate with your teammates during stressful moments? What can you improve?*

- *What are three emotional strengths you bring to your team, and how can you use them to support others?*

_____
_____
_____
_____
_____
_____
_____
_____
_____
_____
_____
_____
_____
_____
_____
_____
_____

CHAPTER 11

"A servant leader must be above reproach, self-controlled, respectable, hospitable, and able to teach."

— *1 Timothy 3:2 (NLT)*

> ***Leadership Beyond Authority:***
> ***Building Trust, Strength, and Vision***

Leadership is more than making decisions or giving orders—it's about inspiring trust, fostering collaboration, and guiding others toward a shared goal. For men, emotional intelligence (EI) is the foundation of effective leadership. It allows you to lead not with authority alone, but with understanding, empathy, and vision. The best leaders aren't just those who know the way forward; they're those who can connect with their teams, understand their needs, and inspire them to rise above challenges.

Think about a leader you admire. Chances are, they didn't just command respect—they earned it through their ability to listen, communicate, and remain composed under pressure. Emotional intelligence helps you do the same by fostering self-awareness, which ensures that your actions align with your values. It also enables self-regulation, so you can respond thoughtfully to challenges instead of reacting impulsively.

Empathy, a cornerstone of EI, allows you to see the struggles and strengths of your team. It gives you the insight to provide encouragement when someone is doubting themselves or to correct someone with grace when they've fallen short. Leadership isn't about perfection—it's about showing up as someone who others can rely on. Emotional intelligence helps you lead with authenticity, allowing others to feel seen, heard, and valued.

> *For men, emotional intelligence (EI) is the foundation of effective leadership.*

As a leader, you set the tone. If you model emotional intelligence—through your resilience, humility, and ability to handle conflict—you create an environment where others feel empowered to grow and thrive. In both your professional and personal life, emotional intelligence isn't just an asset; it's an essential part of becoming the kind of leader who leaves a lasting legacy.

Leadership doesn't begin when you're older, in a high-powered job, or running a business—it starts now. For male youth, emotional intelligence is the foundation for becoming a leader among your peers, in your school, and in your community. Leadership is not about being the loudest or strongest; it's about how you treat others, how you carry yourself, and how you handle challenges.

Imagine you're part of a group project at school, and everyone is stressed because the deadline is near. A leader with emotional intelligence steps up—not to control, but to guide. You might say, "Let's divide the work so everyone feels less overwhelmed," or, "What can I do to help us finish this on time?" Small acts of emotional awareness and empathy show others that you care, earning their trust and respect.

Leadership is also about handling your own emotions. When things don't go your way—whether it's a bad grade, a disagreement with a friend, or a tough loss on the field—your ability to stay calm and think clearly will set you apart. Emotional intelligence gives you the tools to regulate your emotions so you can lead by example. It also helps you resolve conflicts, build friendships, and inspire others to do their best.

Great leaders don't just tell others what to do—they inspire others through their actions. As you grow, focus on building self-awareness, empathy, and communication skills. These are the qualities that will make you not just a good teammate or friend, but a leader others want to follow.

Tools for Men

1. **Daily Self-Reflection**: Spend 5 minutes at the end of each day asking yourself, "How did I lead today? What could I have done differently?"

2. **Empathy Check-Ins**: Make it a habit to ask your team or family members how they're feeling and what support they need.

3. **Conflict Resolution Plan**: Develop a strategy for addressing disagreements calmly, focusing on solutions rather than blame.

Tools for Male Youth

1. **Role Model Study**: Identify a leader you admire and write down the emotional intelligence traits they exhibit. What can you learn from them?

2. **Practice Active Listening**: In conversations, focus on fully understanding the other person before responding.

3. **Group Project Leadership**: Volunteer to take the lead in a team activity or project, using empathy and communication to guide the group.

Reflect & Journal

- *What are three emotional traits I admire in great leaders, and how can I begin to develop those in myself?*

- *Think of a recent conflict or challenge you faced. How did you respond as a leader, and what could you have done differently using emotional intelligence?*

- *What kind of leader do I want to be? What steps can I take today to grow into that role?*

CHAPTER 12

"Life is 10% what happens to you and 90% how you react to it."

— Charles R. Swindoll

> **Mastering The Moment:**
> **Emotional Intelligence In Real Time**

Life doesn't always give you the luxury of preparation. Challenges arise unexpectedly; whether it's a disagreement at work, a sudden family crisis, or even an internal struggle that you didn't see coming. Emotional intelligence in real time is about being present and proactive, not just reactive. It's the ability to apply what you've learned about your emotions, triggers, and responses in the heat of the moment.

Consider a tense meeting where tempers flare, and the conversation veers into conflict. Without emotional intelligence, you might find yourself matching the aggression or shutting down entirely. But with real-time EI, you can pause, assess the situation, and choose a response that defuses rather than escalates. It's not about suppressing how you feel but channeling your emotions constructively.

This ability to stay composed under pressure earns respect, preserves relationships, and helps you make decisions aligned with your values.

> *Emotional intelligence in real time means being able to pause, think, and respond in a way that helps you, rather than hurts you.*

Real-time EI isn't just about conflict; it's about navigating every unpredictable moment. Whether it's comforting a grieving friend, handling unexpected criticism, or adapting to a sudden change in plans, emotional intelligence gives you the tools to face the moment with clarity and resilience. It transforms challenges into opportunities to lead with strength, empathy, and self-awareness.

In the unpredictability of life, real-time emotional intelligence becomes your anchor. It's the skill that ensures you're not ruled by the chaos around you but guided by the wisdom within you. By practicing EI in the moment, you not only handle situations better; you grow through them.

For young men, life can feel like a rollercoaster of emotions, with situations popping up that you didn't expect or know how to handle. Emotional intelligence in real time means being able to pause, think, and respond in a way that helps you, rather than hurts you. It's the difference between letting a bad moment define your day and taking control of your emotions so you can move forward.

Imagine getting into an argument with a friend. The instinct might be to snap back, say something hurtful, or storm off. But real-time EI gives you a better option: pausing and asking yourself, "Why am I feeling this way? What do I want to happen next?" This simple step helps you choose your response instead of letting your emotions take over. It's not about being perfect—it's about staying in control when things feel out of control.

Real-time EI also helps in moments of pressure, like giving a presentation in class or facing disappointment after a tough game. Instead of letting nerves or frustration get the best of you, you can use tools like taking a deep breath or positive self-talk to stay grounded. These small actions may seem simple, but they make a big difference in how you handle life's unpredictable moments.

Tools for Men

1. **Pause and Breathe:** When emotions run high, take three deep breaths before responding. This simple action creates space for clearer thinking.

2. **Ask Yourself Questions:** In the moment, silently ask, "What's the outcome I want here?" or "How can I respond in a way that aligns with my values?"

3. **Anchor to Values:** Identify your core values and let them guide your responses in high-pressure situations.

Tools for Male Youth

1. **Count to Ten:** When you feel angry or frustrated, count to ten before speaking or acting. This helps prevent impulsive reactions.

2. **Buddy Check:** When faced with a tough situation, talk to a trusted friend, teacher, or mentor to process your emotions.

3. **Journal the Moment:** After handling an unexpected situation, write about what happened, how you felt, and what you learned from it.

EMOTIONAL INTELLIGENCE

Cracking the Code for Men & Male Youth

Reflect & Journal

- *When faced with uncertainty, do you react with fear or strategy? How can you shift your mindset?*

- *What's one painful transition in your life that ultimately made you stronger? What did you learn?*

- *How can you use emotional intelligence to trust the process instead of resisting change?*

CHAPTER 13

"A fool gives full vent to his anger, but a wise man quietly holds it back."

— Proverbs 29:11 (NLT)

What Does God Say About Emotional Intelligence?

Emotional intelligence is not a modern concept, it's deeply rooted in biblical principles. Throughout scripture, we see examples of wisdom, self-control, empathy, and discernment—all of which are key components of EI. The Bible teaches us that wisdom begins with understanding (Proverbs 4:7), and part of that understanding is recognizing our emotions and how they shape our thoughts and actions. The ability to manage emotions wisely isn't just a personal advantage; it's a reflection of God's wisdom working in us. EI allows us to respond to life's challenges with grace, love, patience, and discernment, rather than reacting out of impulse.

Jesus was not only the Son of God but also the greatest example of emotional intelligence ever displayed. He showed self-awareness in His moments of solitude, knowing when He needed time alone to pray and recharge. He demonstrated self-regulation when confronted by the Pharisees, never allowing anger to control His actions, even when falsely accused. He exemplified deep empathy, weeping with those who mourned (John 11:35) and healing the brokenhearted. His motivation was unwavering, knowing that His purpose on earth was greater than temporary suffering. And His social skills allowed Him to lead, correct, and teach with authority yet gentleness. As men, we often react instead of responding, allowing emotions like pride, frustration, or impatience to dictate our behavior. But when we look to Jesus, we see the power of responding with wisdom, grace, and understanding. Emotional intelligence is not about weakness, it's about strength under control, just as Jesus displayed in every moment of His life.

As a young man, you might often feel like your emotions are all over the place; anger, frustration, sadness, or even excitement that turns into recklessness. The world may tell you that real strength is in hiding your emotions or ignoring them altogether,

> *Emotional intelligence is not a modern concept, it's deeply rooted in biblical principles.*

but God teaches something different. Proverbs 29:11 says, **"A fool gives full vent to his anger, but a wise man quietly holds it back."** This doesn't mean bottling up emotions but learning to manage them in a way that honors God. You don't have to pretend you're okay when you're not, but you can practice pausing, praying, and asking God for wisdom before reacting. Emotional intelligence is your ability to recognize what you feel, understand why you feel it, and respond in a way that leads to growth rather than regret.

Many young men struggle with conflict, whether it's arguments with parents, disagreements with friends, or feeling disrespected. The Bible teaches us that how we respond in these moments matters. James 1:19-20 says, **"Understand this, my dear brothers and sisters: You must all be quick to listen, slow to speak, and slow to get angry. Human anger does not produce the righteousness God desires."** This is emotional intelligence in action. Instead of immediately lashing out when someone offends you, practice listening first. Instead of responding with anger, take a moment to ask yourself, "What would Jesus do in this situation?" Choosing patience, kindness, and wisdom in your relationships will set you apart as a leader among your peers. The way you handle emotions today will shape the kind of man you become tomorrow.

Tools for Men

1. **The Pause & Pray Method** – Before reacting in anger, frustration, or disappointment, pause and take a moment to pray for wisdom and discernment.

2. **Biblical Emotional Check-In** – Identify an emotion you struggle with (anger, impatience, fear) and find a scripture that speaks to that feeling. Meditate on it daily.

3. **Spiritual Journaling** – At the end of each week, reflect on one emotional challenge you faced and how you handled it. What would God say about your response?

Tools for Male Youth

1. **WWJD (What Would Jesus Do?) Exercise** – Before reacting to a tough situation, ask yourself how Jesus would respond and try to model His behavior.

2. **Daily Scripture Reminder** – Choose one verse about patience, wisdom, or self-control and repeat it throughout your day.

3. **Empathy Challenge** – Try to put yourself in someone else's shoes before making a judgment or reacting emotionally. This will help you build deeper relationships.

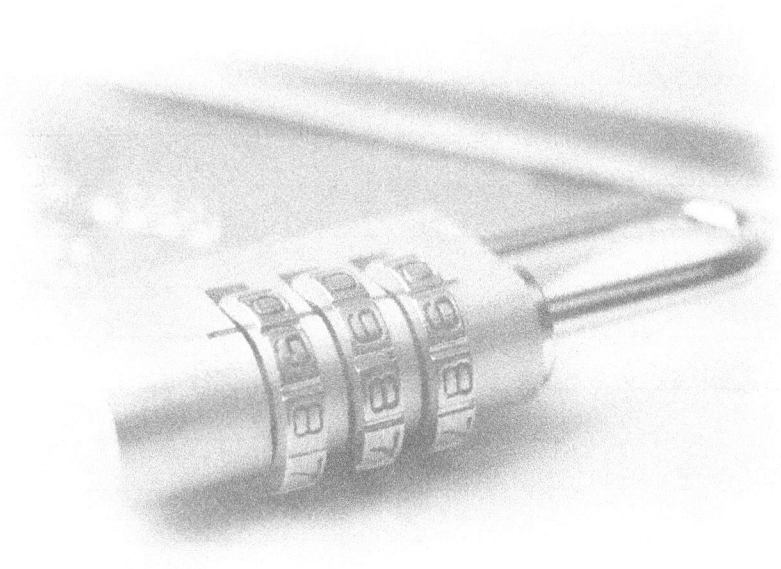

Reflect & Journal

- *Which emotions do I struggle with the most, and how can I invite God into those areas of my life?*

- *How does my emotional intelligence impact my relationships with others and with God?*

- *What is one example from Jesus' life where He demonstrated emotional intelligence, and how can I apply that lesson to my own life?*

CHAPTER 14

"You don't have to control your thoughts. You just have to stop letting them control you."

– Dan Millman

> **Emotional Intelligence Turns Mental Health Into Mental Wealth**

Breaking the Cycle of Emotional Suppression & Mental Struggles

For far too long, men have been conditioned to believe that suppressing their emotions is a sign of strength. We're taught to "suck it up," to "push through," and to handle our struggles in silence. But what happens when the weight of unspoken pain, unresolved anger, and buried stress becomes too heavy? It manifests in ways we don't always recognize, short tempers, anxiety, disconnection, self-sabotage, and even physical health issues.

The reality is that many men are trapped in cycles of emotional suppression without realizing that these habits are directly affecting their mental health. Depression doesn't always look like sadness; it can look like irritability, detachment, or even an overcommitment to work to avoid dealing with emotions. Anxiety isn't always panic attacks; sometimes, it's the constant pressure to meet impossible expectations or a fear of failure that keeps us up at night. Emotional intelligence is the bridge that allows us to recognize, process, and navigate these struggles in a way that brings healing, rather than destruction.

Men who develop emotional intelligence understand that self-awareness isn't weakness, it's wisdom. They learn that emotions are signals, not enemies. Instead of numbing their pain with work, alcohol, or unhealthy distractions, they learn how to face it, process it, and heal from it. Emotional intelligence teaches us that seeking help isn't a sign of failure, but a demonstration of courage. Whether that help comes from therapy, mentorship, faith, or a brotherhood of like-minded men, acknowledging that you need support is one of the greatest acts of self-leadership you can take.

> *Depression doesn't always look like sadness; it can look like irritability, detachment, or even an overcommitment to work to avoid dealing with emotions.*

If you want to improve your mental health, you have to start by improving how you manage your emotions, process your pain, and release what's been weighing you down. Emotional intelligence won't remove challenges from your life, but it will give you the tools to navigate them without losing yourself in the process.

Learning Emotional Intelligence Early to Protect Your Mental Well-Being

For young men and male youth, emotions can feel overwhelming, especially when no one has ever taught you what to do with them. You might not always recognize it, but your emotions shape how you react in school, in sports, in friendships, and in family dynamics. Without emotional intelligence, it's easy to lash out in anger, shut down when you're hurt, or feel lost when things don't go as planned.

Think about this: How often do you feel like no one understands what you're going through? Maybe you've had moments where you felt frustrated but didn't know how to explain it, so you just got mad instead. Or times where you felt hurt but decided to laugh it off because showing emotion made you feel weak. This pattern of hiding emotions can lead to stress, loneliness, and even mental health struggles like anxiety and depression.

Emotional intelligence gives you a different path. It teaches you how to recognize what you feel and why you feel it, so you can respond instead of react. It helps you communicate what's going on inside without feeling ashamed or misunderstood. Instead of bottling up emotions until they explode, you learn how to express them in a way that allows others to support you, not judge you.

If you're a student-athlete, an artist, or simply a young man trying to figure things out, understanding your emotions will give you an advantage in every area of life. It will help you build stronger friendships, work through frustration without losing control, and take care of your mental well-being before it spirals into something unmanageable. Learning this now will prepare you for a future where you are not controlled by emotions but in control of them.

Tools for Men

1. **Daily Emotional Check-Ins** – Ask yourself: *What am I feeling right now? Why? How is this affecting my actions?*

2. **Journaling for Clarity** – Write out your thoughts to release emotions, recognize patterns, and find solutions.

3. **Therapy or Mentorship** – Having someone to process emotions with helps you gain perspective and heal.

4. **Mindfulness & Stress Reduction** – Practices like deep breathing, meditation, or faith-based reflection can calm your mind.

5. **Building a Support Network** – Find men who understand your struggles and create a space for open conversations.

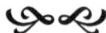

Tools for Male Youth

1. **Name Your Emotions** – Instead of saying *"I'm just mad,"* identify *why*—are you frustrated? Hurt? Disappointed?

2. **Talk to Someone You Trust** – Whether it's a coach, mentor, or friend, opening up about struggles prevents isolation.

3. **Use Physical Activity as an Outlet** – Sports, working out, or even walking can help relieve stress in a healthy way.

4. **Practice Positive Self-Talk** – Replace thoughts like *"I'll never be good enough"* with *"I'm still learning and growing."*

5. **Pause Before Reacting** – When you're upset, take five deep breaths before you respond. It can prevent regretful reactions.

EMOTIONAL INTELLIGENCE

Cracking the Code for Men & Male Youth

Reflect & Journal

- *What are some emotions you have avoided or ignored in the past? How did this impact you?*

- *How can Emotional Intelligence help you better manage your mental health?*

- *What steps will you take to improve your emotional awareness and mental well-being moving forward?*

_____
_____
_____
_____
_____
_____
_____
_____
_____
_____

Mental health is not about being perfect or always having it together. It's about knowing how to take care of yourself, how to manage your emotions, and how to reach out for support when you need it. Emotional intelligence is your tool, your shield, and your strategy for maintaining a strong, healthy mind.

You have two choices: You can let your emotions control you, or you can learn to control them. The decision you make will shape the rest of your life. Choose growth. Choose self-awareness. Choose emotional intelligence.

CHAPTER 15

> **The Final Chapter, EI The First Choice:**
> **Making Emotional Intelligence Your Way of Life**

Congratulations. If you've made it this far, you've done something that most people never do, you've chosen to invest in your emotional intelligence, your mental well-being, and ultimately, your future. This book wasn't just about learning new information, it was about equipping you with a new way to see yourself, your emotions, and your ability to navigate life.

You now hold something powerful: the ability to respond instead of react, to lead instead of follow, and to build instead of break. But knowledge without action is meaningless. Now, it's time to apply everything you've learned.

> *Mental health is not about being perfect or always having it together.*

The real work starts the moment you close this book. How you choose to implement Emotional Intelligence (EI) will shape your relationships, your career, your leadership, your mental health, and your ability to impact those around you.

So, what's next? How do you take everything you've learned and make it a way of life? This final chapter is your roadmap.

Making EI a Daily Habit

Emotional intelligence isn't something you "use" every now and then—it's something you embody every single day. It's in the way you handle stress, communicate with others, process setbacks, and push yourself to grow.

Here's how you can integrate EI into your life daily:

1. Self-Awareness: Make Reflection a Routine

- Every morning, ask yourself: "How am I feeling today?"

- Every night, ask yourself: "How did I handle my emotions today? What can I improve?"

- Journal at least once a week to track your emotions, reactions, and growth.

- **Real-Life Application for Men:** Before responding to a stressful email, a frustrating conversation, or a difficult decision, pause. Ask yourself: *"What am I feeling, and why? What's the best way to respond?"*

- **Real-Life Application for Male Youth:** If you get a bad grade, miss a shot in a game, or feel disrespected by someone, before reacting in anger or frustration, pause. Ask yourself: *"What's really making me upset? Is there a better way to handle this?"*

---

2. Self-Regulation: Control Your Reactions, Don't Let Them Control You

- Develop a "cool-off strategy"—count to 10, take a deep breath, go for a walk before reacting.

- When you feel emotions rising, ask yourself: "Is my reaction helping or hurting the situation?"

- Learn to sit with your emotions instead of running from them.

- **Real-Life Application for Men:** The next time you're in a heated conversation with a coworker, partner, or family member, instead of reacting with frustration, take a step back and think before responding.

- **Real-Life Application for Male Youth:** If a teammate, teacher, or friend makes you angry, instead of lashing out, take a deep breath, walk away if needed, and come back to the conversation with a clear mind.

> ### 3. Motivation: Set Goals That Align with Your Values
>
> - Define your "why"—why do you want to be emotionally intelligent? What kind of man do you want to be?
>
> - Set personal goals that challenge you emotionally and mentally.
>
> - Track your progress and celebrate small wins—growth takes time.

- **Real-Life Application for Men:** Write down a goal related to your emotional growth (ex: "I will communicate better with my partner," "I will manage my stress better at work"). Revisit this goal weekly.

- **Real-Life Application for Male Youth:** Pick one area of self-improvement (ex: "I will respond calmly when I feel disrespected," "I will focus on schoolwork without getting discouraged"). Hold yourself accountable.

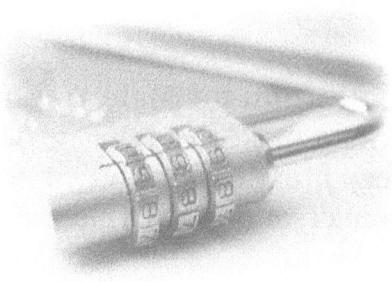

> **4. Empathy: Build Stronger Relationships by Understanding Others**
>
> - Practice active listening—instead of waiting to talk, focus on understanding.
>
> - Put yourself in others' shoes before judging or reacting.
>
> - Ask more questions—people want to feel heard.

- **Real-Life Application for Men:** The next time someone you care about is upset, instead of offering advice or trying to fix it, simply listen. Let them know you hear them.

- **Real-Life Application for Male Youth:** If a friend is struggling, don't make it about you—ask them how they feel, what they need, and how you can support them.

5. Social Skills: Communicate with Confidence and Clarity

- Master nonverbal cues—eye contact, posture, tone of voice.

- Learn how to express emotions without aggression or avoidance.

- Surround yourself with people who challenge and support your growth.

- **Real-Life Application for Men:** Next time you need to express how you feel, use "I" statements instead of blaming. Example: *"I feel overwhelmed when I don't get support,"* instead of *"You never help me!"*

- **Real-Life Application for Male Youth:** If you're upset with a coach, teacher, or parent, express your feelings clearly, not aggressively. Example: *"I feel frustrated because I worked hard and didn't get the result I wanted."*

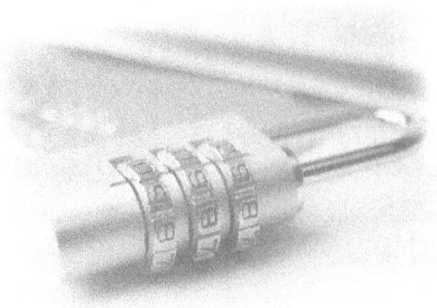

FINAL MESSAGE

> *The Legacy of Emotional Intelligence*

Every choice you make from this moment forward will either strengthen or weaken your emotional intelligence. The question is, will you use what you've learned?

You have a responsibility—not just to yourself, but to those around you. The way you handle your emotions, communicate, and lead will impact your family, your relationships, and the next generation of men who are watching you.

Emotional intelligence is not about being perfect. It's about being aware, being intentional, and being willing to grow.

The world does not need more men who suppress their emotions, explode under pressure, or shut down in hard times. It needs more men who can regulate their emotions, lead with empathy, and build strong relationships.

This is your moment to break cycles. To set a new standard. To become a man who leads himself first, so he can lead others well.

As you close this book, remember:

- Your emotional intelligence will determine the quality of your relationships, your success, and your mental well-being.

- You don't just read about emotional intelligence—you live it, you practice it, and you make it your way of life.

- The work doesn't stop here. This is only the beginning.

Now, go apply what you've learned. Your future, your relationships, and your peace of mind depend on it.

EMOTIONAL INTELLIGENCE

Cracking the Code for Men & Male Youth

Reflect & Journal

- *What is one emotional intelligence skill you've grown in since reading this book? How has it changed the way you handle life?*

- *Which area of emotional intelligence (self-awareness, self-regulation, motivation, empathy, social skills) do you need to work on most? What's one action step you'll take this week?*

- *What kind of man do you want to become because of your emotional intelligence growth? How will you hold yourself accountable?*

_____

_____

_____

_____

_____

_____

_____

_____

_____

_____

_____

_____

_____

_____

_____

_____

**This book gave you the tools.
Now it's time to build.**

Your growth doesn't stop here. Keep learning, keep leading, and most importantly, keep showing up for yourself.

EMOTIONAL INTELLIGENCE

Cracking the Code for Men & Male Youth

FROM THE AUTHOR

As I bring this book to a close, I want to take a moment to thank you. Not just for reading, but for embarking on this journey of self-discovery and growth. Writing this book has been more than an opportunity to share knowledge; it has been a reflection of my own journey with emotional intelligence. There have been moments in my life where my lack of self-awareness, my inability to regulate my emotions, or my failure to empathize deeply with others cost me relationships, opportunities, and peace of mind. I've learned, often the hard way, that emotional intelligence is not just a skill; it's a way of living, leading, and loving.

I remember a time when I let anger get the best of me in a personal situation. My reaction was immediate and fueled by frustration, and though I felt justified in the moment, I quickly realized the damage it caused to the trust and respect I had built with those close to me. It wasn't until I reflected on that moment, sought understanding, and took accountability for my actions that I was able to mend what had been broken. That experience taught me the power of pausing, reflecting, and responding with intention, lessons that have now reshaped how I show up as a leader, husband, father, and friend.

For me, emotional intelligence has been a process of growth, not perfection. There are days when I get it right and days when I fall short, but I've come to understand that the journey itself is where the transformation happens. My hope is that this book has provided you with the tools to begin your own journey, to navigate life with clarity, and to connect with others in ways that bring meaning and purpose.

To the men and male youth reading this: know that emotional intelligence is not about weakness; it's about courage. It's the courage to face your emotions, to acknowledge your flaws, and to choose growth even when it's hard. It's about showing up fully—not just for others, but for yourself.

As you take the lessons of this book and put them into action, remember that the impact of your growth doesn't stop with you. Every time you choose understanding over judgment, vulnerability over silence, or patience over anger, you create a ripple effect that touches everyone around you. Your growth becomes a gift—not just to yourself, but to your family, your community, and the generations that follow.

Thank you for allowing me to be a part of your journey. Writing this book has been one of the most meaningful experiences of my life, and it is my sincere hope that it inspires you to live with intention, embrace emotional intelligence, and leave a legacy of connection and impact. This is not the end of the journey, it's the beginning.

Let's keep growing, together, one step at a time.

With gratitude,
Clarence J. Grant, Jr.

GLOSSARY

Emotional Intelligence: the ability to recognize, understand, and manage your own emotions while effectively navigating and understanding the emotions of others

Self-Awareness: understanding your emotions, strengths, weaknesses, values, and triggers. It's one of the foundational components of emotional intelligence allowing you to make informed decisions and respond thoughtfully

Self-Regulation: managing your emotions, especially in stressful or triggering situations, and behaving in ways that align with your values

Motivation: the driving force behind every achievement

Empathy: the ability to step outside your own perspective and truly understand the emotions and experiences of others

Social Skills: the glue that holds relationships together, both personally and professionally

Notes

Notes

Notes

Notes

Notes

Notes

Notes

Notes

Notes

www.ingramcontent.com/pod-product-compliance
Lightning Source LLC
Chambersburg PA
CBHW071721020426
42333CB00017B/2347